In Pursuit of Grit

In Pursuit of Grit

5 Ways to Transform Your Mind, Develop Your
Character and Get the Body You Desire

DARRELL WILLIAMS, CCS

ISBN-13: 9780692890837
ISBN-10: 0692890831
Library of Congress Control Number: 2017918817
Darrell Williams, East Elmhurst, NY

The methods described within this book are the author's personal
thoughts. They are not intended to be a definitive set of instructions
for this project. You may discover other methods and materials to
accomplish the same end results.

To contact the author visit our website at www.thegritregime.com

Bible scripture taken from the New King James Version (NKJV®).
Copyright © 1982 by Thomas Nelson. All rights reserved.

To my amazing parents for raising me and directing me to the right path

Your hardship and sacrifice throughout the years were not in vain. I cherish every heartache and pain it took for you to mold me into the person I am today. I love you both deeply.

To my seventeen siblings

Individually, you all mean more to me than your minds could ever fathom. Each one of you has gifts and talents I could only dream of having. Being with you, I am constantly reminded to be a better son, a better brother, and a better person. Thank you! I love you all!

Contents

Your Free Gift

As part of your journey to improve your willpower and the pursuit of grit, I have sent you a free seventy-seven-day calendar to go along with your seventy-seven days of creating a new habit. In addition, I have created a grit manifesto so that you can be reminded of why you're on this journey and why it's not an option to give up. Go to the following links to get your free accountability calendar and your grit manifesto:

Calendar—https://roguegrit.lpages.co/thegritcalendar/

Manifesto—https://roguegrit.lpages.co/thegritmanifesto

Acknowledgments

Special thanks to Paul Hertzog, Eric Isles, Elsie Morgan, Teresa Silversmith, Timothy Trammell, Beverly Weeks, Hasan Williams, Julia Williams, Qiydaar Williams, and Fleur Marie Vaz, my editor from Malaysia.

During the process of writing this book, I received invaluable help and support from my amazing wife throughout this incredible journey. Simmone without you, this road would have been difficult to navigate on my own. Thank you for your patience, your knowledge, and your advice. You are deeply appreciated.

Introduction

You're probably asking yourself, "What is grit? How could it help me with my exercise regimen or even my everyday life?"

By definition, *grit* is firmness of mind or spirit, unyielding courage in the face of hardship or danger.[1] Grit is vital for cultivating a strong character, as it allows you to persevere through life's obstacles, whether you are pursuing short- or long-term goals. It gives you the tenacity not to wave the white flag once opposition comes. By pursuing grit, you accept the fact that you are exposing yourself to constant discomfort. This is not a bad thing, however, because grit strengthens your mind to adapt to such pain and subsequently prepares you to better face hardships along your path.

I am sure that, at various points in your life, there were periods in which you went through some type of hardship to accomplish a particular goal. Maybe you are struggling to overcome a certain obstacle at this very moment as you read this book. Perhaps you have an important exam coming up and you need to buckle down and study. Your pain is certainly disciplining you to study for hours on end to achieve the short-term goal of getting an excellent grade. The power of grit could help you make the necessary sacrifices to meet your target.

In the same way, grit could help you in your exercise regimen. Grit enables you to be mentally prepared to accomplish your fitness goals. Without it, you would slow down once the discomfort of pain arrives. Pain is something we do not desire by nature. But grit makes the pain tolerable and gives you the persistence to push through, knowing the pain is part of the process of creating the body you desperately desire. Soon the pain will not be a factor to avoid because you begin to see it as a positive sign you are achieving your ideal visual image. Eventually you start to embrace the pain, knowing that, in the process of developing your physique, you also mature your character. Never again will pain deter you from the gym.

You are probably wondering what motivated me to write a book on grit. Well, allow me to tell you. This book is actually a testimony of my life from the initial doubts and struggles I faced to the hardship I gracefully embraced because I knew that developing strong willpower would help me through my trials. But I realized having a strong willpower wasn't enough. I had to go and pursue something greater: grit.

To be frank, one of the main reasons I wrote this book was my diagnosis of attention deficit hyperactivity disorder, or ADHD, back in March 2016. Behavioral and cognitive symptoms, such as hyperactivity, inattention, disorganization, and impulsivity, characterize ADHD. The symptoms must be severe and cause clinically significant impairment persistently in multiple domains of an individual's life in order to warrant a diagnosis.[2]

This news was a dreadful blow to me. Strangely enough, once I finally received the doctor's report, I was actually quite relieved. I knew all along that something wasn't right during my adolescent and young adult life, but I started to become more self-aware as an adult and really evaluated myself seriously. I was relieved because I was able to put a label to the many years of disorganization, procrastination, total lack of time management skills, and so on.

In this battle with ADHD, I am constantly at war within myself because of how it affects my mind and body. One of the most common signs of this disorder is the tendency to start a task and not finish it. I have to constantly fight against ADHD hijacking my mind and getting me to lose track of the task and be distracted by something else. But I am determined to finish this book in my personal quest for grit.

Ever since I was a teenager, I have been drawn to physical fitness. Competition was the driving force. I remember having push-up and sit-up contests with my older brothers, always eager to push myself so I could beat them, being the younger sibling. That's one of the reasons I developed a strong will. As a young man, this passion for fitness and a love for the gym continued and helped me strengthen my willpower.

But what's the point of having a strong will just to be hindered by disorganization, inability to prioritize, and procrastination due to my attention disorder? It's true that I had the will to be fairly consistent at the gym and to work toward a decent physique. I definitely had the will to challenge myself and surpass what my body thought was not possible. On the other hand, I was not consistent in my meal planning or the process of planning my exercise sessions in order to get the necessary rest to replenish my muscles. This was the adverse effect that ADHD had on my fitness regime.

In Pursuit of Grit

One day, I looked at myself in the mirror, and I wondered how I was supposed to achieve my ideal physique if I couldn't maintain consistency. How could I combat and master ADHD with my dull tool of willpower alone? How could I achieve a productive life if all I could do was start up a task but never follow it through? That was the day I decided to put on my coat, tighten my bootstraps, and prepare to go into the "storm of discomfort" in the pursuit of grit. I resolved to reclaim my vital keys from being robbed by ADHD—the keys to normal brain functionality, the keys to my life. It was all within arm's reach, but it would not be easy.

Are you ready to come with me on this venture to get back our keys in the pursuit of grit? Let's get back to the gym scenario. Let's address the issue of making excuses.

Are you sick and tired of signing up for a gym membership and only going for the first two weeks in January? Or are you habitually breaking your clean eating diet by having countless cheat meals throughout the week? We have many reasons why we excuse ourselves for not keeping to our fitness goals. The more excuses we give, the further we move from our goals. You don't want to reach your sixties and ask yourself, "What have I ever accomplished?" when you aim to be the best version of yourself.

But guess what? I have great news for you. What if I told you that change comes from within? It starts in your mind. They say abs are created in the kitchen, but I say they are wrong. Strong abs, like everything else, starts in the mind.

I can help you accomplish your goals. But first we just have to get over excuses like:

- "I feel self-conscious about my physique."
- "I fear others will criticize me."
- "I am my own worst critic; I judge myself harshly."
- "I didn't see any results, so I just stopped going."
- "I'm too tired to go to the gym."
- "It's too crowded."
- "It's a rainy day."
- "I've been hitting the gym, but I can't work out with a sore body."

By reading this step-by-step guide, you're actually taking the first step toward improving your willpower and pursuing grit. So give yourself a pat on the back, because you are definitely on the right track to victory!

I know you're probably asking yourself, "I've been doing everything in my power to carve out a better body in the gym. How will this book change my thinking and my life?" Well, I was once in your shoes. I used to make all the excuses in the book to avoid going to the gym. I now realize these excuses came from disorganization, procrastination, lack of grit, and not knowing I had a mental disorder.

But gradually my life started to change. I reset my mental apparatus. I discovered that whatever I do, especially if it pertains to working out, starts in the mind. I realized I had a flawed perception of things. I wasn't working out my "mental muscle." If I wanted to see drastic changes in my life, I had to strengthen that mental muscle.

In the process, I discovered five secret strategies that I want to share with you. The first strategy is *self-affirmation*. Self-affirmation allows you to replace any negative self-talk with a positive affirmation. The second strategy is *the power of the mind*, which is the will to control your mind to desire something that your brain is not naturally designed to do. The third strategy is *the pleasure principle versus the reality principle*. This battle reminds you of the constant war within yourself so that you won't operate in an impulsive state of immediate gratification but under the control of delayed gratification. The fourth strategy is *the visionary's reconstruction*. This strategy enables you to change your vision of an outcome to produce a positive emotion to help drive a desirable result. The final strategy is *the mind's comfort zone*. This strategy forces your mind to be in an uncomfortable environment, such as envisioning your fears, so that you familiarize your mind with your fears to the extent that the fears no longer cause discomfort. You can apply these strategies to your life to improve your consistency, your discipline, your will-power, and your grit for the gym. You can reach your goals in just seventy-seven days—not just goals for inside the gym but also for outside the gym, in your own life.

*Taking the path less followed is hard
because you walk alone sometimes,
but you have the inner strength
to do it. Not everyone does.*

Teresa Silversmith, MBA,
RHIT, CCS, C-CDI

One

Self-Affirmation: The Too-Tired Excuse

Death and life are in the power
of the tongue, And those who
love it will eat its fruit.

—Proverbs 18:21

I t's finally five o'clock on a Friday evening. You're walking to the time clock to punch out with a sense of urgency. You want to get out of there as fast as possible. You've come to realize that you're just too exhausted from a long week, and the one thing you want to do is go straight home and watch TV. The last place you want to be at is the gym.

1

As you're getting into your car, you're still deciding whether to go to the gym or home to relax. You're completely aware that your house is just five miles away and the gym is actually ten. On the road to uncertainty, you start to yawn, making your eyes water, which inevitably leads to the decision to take Exit 7, the way home.

Okay, you finally made your decision. Are you satisfied? Are you okay with investing so much time and effort in your nine-to-five job yet neglecting to invest in yourself in what would have taken only an hour out of your day? Can you sleep at night knowing that, week after week, you've made the conscious decision to go home and place yourself on the back burner, while the company you work for is getting the best out of you? What about your dream of a healthier body or your goal of losing those extra pounds? How are you going to alleviate the stress at work if you're constantly too tired to invest in yourself and your health?

What happened to your vision of having a muscular physique and better self-esteem? Do I sense a case of dreams deferred simply because you're just too tired? If something needs to be done, are you going to delay it because you don't have the energy? What a sad-lived life, where nothing is ever accomplished and procrastination takes over simply because the too-tired excuse has taken you on a perpetual diversion via Exit 7!

Self-Affirmation

But I have good news. Self-affirmation can turn things around. The words of self-affirmation spoken out loud will travel into the core of your being. These affirmations will tell your subconscious what you should believe about yourself, and the change will start happening from within. But ingrained negative thoughts and negative confessions can resist this process. If an unwholesome belief has become entrenched in your subconscious mind, then it can override a positive affirmation, even if you aren't aware of it. This is why positive affirmations alone do not seem to work for many people. Their negative thought patterns are so strong that they cancel out the effect of the positive statements. So how can we add more muscle to an affirmation so that it has the power to override our negativity?

Neurolinguistic Programming (NLP)

The underlying strategy to add muscle to your self-affirmations is neurolinguistic programming (NLP),[3] which is based on the belief that although we observe the natural world through our senses, these impressions are filtered through the lens of our belief system, values, and attitudes. So there is the objective world, and there is the world that is viewed though our subjective experiences.

NLP goes on to posit that we have the ability to alter our reality by the way we choose to think, feel, communicate, and behave. The emotions we choose to portray during particular episodes will, over time, influence our view of the world and ourselves.

Let's analyze the term neurolinguistic programming. "Neuro" refers to the mind. "Linguistic" refers to language. And "programming" involves behavior. With the help of your five senses, your mind allows you to perceive the world from your individual perspective. The language is your communication with yourself, people, and real-life scenarios. The programming is your outward behavior in response to your perception of the world, other people, and situations.

Imagine stepping out into a dull and gloomy day. Do you have to feel gloomy? No, you can modify your response to your environment to feel good on the inside because you have set your mind on being productive today. In this way, you can modify your perception of yourself and the things around you to create a desirable outcome. All this adds to your personal growth. By doing so, you are initiating a change in the way you think, talk, and react to your own impulses and your surroundings. This is called reprogramming.

NLP helps us to reprogram our mind away from a negative mind-set. The basic method it advocates is to speak positive affirmations out loud and consistently for about five minutes.[4] Practice your self-affirmations three times a day—morning, midday, and evening—as if you were taking a doctor's prescription. An ideal time would be when you're putting on your makeup or shaving so that you can look at yourself in the mirror as you repeat the positive declarations.

As you say these words, you are slowly but surely speaking life into your innermost being. You are freeing your mind of the negative experiences accumulated over the years that were deposited into your subconscious and that held you captive. You have the keys to come out of that prison of the mind. Your positive affirmations, confessed several times each day, are both the tools and the strategy for you to break out into a vibrant, new self.

One important technique of reprogramming to alter our negative self-talk is to switch from present to past tense. You put the negative experiences into the past and the positive experiences into the present. Consider these scenarios:

- Instead of saying, "I tend to procrastinate every time I think about the gym," say, "In the past, I would procrastinate about going to the gym, but now I just go without thinking about it."
- Instead of saying, "I have cravings for chocolate whenever I am depressed," say, "In the past, I had

cravings for chocolate whenever I was depressed. But now I have overcome depression and can control my eating."

See what's happening? By switching your negative statements from present to past tense, you are training your mind and body to view your negative mind-set as a thing of the past and to view your present as brimming with possibilities.

The battle for the mind is so crucial that Proverbs 4:23 warns us to carefully guard our thought life. "Keep your heart with all diligence, For out it spring the issues of life."

Not only our thought life but also our tongues need to come under strict control because they can deal life or death to their users. "Death and life are in the power of the tongue, And those who love it will eat its fruit" (Proverbs 18:2).

Drawing from these vital truths, NLP encourages us to strengthen our self-affirmations by strengthening our thought life. The more we implement positive self-affirmations, the stronger we become mentally. The more we think positive thoughts, the more we speak positively. "A good man out of the good treasure of his heart brings forth good; and an evil man out of the evil treasure of his heart brings forth evil. For out of the abundance of the heart his mouth speaks" (Luke 6:45). What we think and feel forms our emotions and establishes our beliefs and attitudes. So when every part of the thinking-speaking process is positive and life-giving, with repetition over time, we can confidently look toward greater self-assurance with no room for self-doubt.

For example, here is a typical scenario without the intervention of NLP:

You're driving during rush-hour traffic and conclude it's going to take you hours to get home. You sigh and mutter under your breath, "If only I hadn't taken this route!" Someone rolls down his car window to let you know there was an accident a quarter of a mile ahead. This news agitates you further. You start to get frustrated and honk the horn. You accidently press on the gas and hit the car in front of you.

Here is the altered scenario with the intervention of NLP combined with self-affirmations:

You're driving during rush-hour traffic and guess it may probably take you some time to get home. So you start to play soothing music to relax your mind. You make these affirmations, "Well, there's no reason to be in a rush to get home. As long as I get home safely, I'm fine." You discover that there's been an accident ahead from the neighboring car's announcement, and you keep your cool and refrain from reacting in anger.

In short, the life-generating words of self-affirmation are going to strengthen your belief system and dismantle your self-doubt and wayward thoughts. This results in building your grit and willpower. In the following chapters, I will share four other secrets of building your character. Self-affirmation is the glue that binds the four concepts all together.

Now that we know the value of self-affirmation, let's return to the opening scene where you are walking to the time clock to punch out of work. Of course, by this hour of the day, you're going to be tired, no doubt about it. But you have to put the thought of "too tired" in a mental hold so that you can focus on your real goal, the workout.

As you're walking, tired and beat, to that time clock, you will yourself to stand up to negate and overpower the feeling of weariness by making these self-affirmations:

- "I am worth investing time in."
- "I'm tired, but my will for my health and my goals is stronger than my feelings."

- "I will not allow my emotions to rob me of my dreams."
- "It's Friday evening. I'd rather go home to relax, but I want to place myself first and go to the gym. I can rest on the weekend."

The repetition of NLP and self-affirmations are the most effective ways to form a new habit for developing self-belief, self-encouragement, and grit. But you must be realistic. Unrealistic expectations of the time frame to develop a good habit can lead you to be frustrated and to give up during the waiting phase. Some people may have heard that habits take twenty-one days to form. This belief is not actually proven with scientific evidence. Current research has found that most people plateau at around sixty-six days after the first day. Therefore, it may be helpful to expect the new habit to be established through daily repetition after ten weeks.[5]

Research also finds that people are reassured to learn that repeating the behavior gets progressively easier, so they only have to maintain their motivation until the habit is formed. In short, working intentionally on a new behavior for two to three months increases the chance of the behavior becoming second nature.

As for me, my willpower was strong enough for my fitness regimen, but I still struggled with the effects ADHD had on my total management ability. I was able to push myself to lift a high volume of weight by adding more weight to the bar after each set was over. But it was a major task for me to plan out my workout routine prior to going to the gym. I recall going to the gym for months without writing down my exercise plan for the week and sometimes for the month. This is how ADHD continued to push back on my progress. I had to intentionally implement the use of self-affirmation to strengthen the areas I was particularly weak at: organization, consistency, and acquiring the grit I needed to execute my plan. I needed these attributes to be able to formulate a blueprint of my workout for the month and to be diligent enough to attentively view my plan on a daily basis.

In the process, I learned to make the following self-affirmations:

- "I will create a monthly workout plan for the month and view it daily to create the body I've always dreamt of."
- "As my organization skills improve, I will be more consistent in the gym and in my personal life."
- "Regardless of how many times I experience pain and struggles in the gym or life, I must acquire the grit I need for mental and physical development."

In Pursuit of Grit

I therefore purposefully exposed myself to this unfamiliar realm, the world of grit. Admittedly, it has often been extremely uncomfortable combating this unfortunate mental disorder, but I continue to press on to enhance my organization, consistency, and pursuit of grit. I often have to force my own will to go against the way ADHD had wired my brain. At first, the affirmations I made sounded like empty words, but gradually they became alive as I heard them spoken out loud, and I began to think in accordance with my words.

Over time, my positive confessions started to produce results—a more organized, consistent, and stable self. Confronting ADHD is still an uphill battle, and I have no option but to continually rewire and take charge of my mind till it reaches its optimal state. I continue to pursue grit!

I would encourage you to make your positive affirmations out loud for a little over two months, especially when you're tired and tempted to take the easy route. I promise you will see definite results. Repetition is the key. You have to get the escape route of Exit 7 out of your thinking pattern and reprogram it by unleashed secret power of self-affirmation. In a matter of weeks, you'll be taking Exit 10 to the gym without even a second thought!

For the first two weeks, concentrate on practicing self-affirmation accompanied by neurolinguistic programming. Implement this in your everyday life so that you can begin the process of creating a new and positive habit.

Two

The Power of the Mind: The Inconsistency Excuse

*And do not be conformed to this world,
but be transformed by the renewing of your
mind, that may prove what is that good
and acceptable and perfect will of God.*

—Romans 12:2

Are you a person who frequently starts something but doesn't finish it? Every time a good idea comes to mind, do you suddenly drop the task you were just working on and move on to the next thing? As you look back in time, do you see a vast array of unfinished tasks and projects that you've neglected because something new came along? This scattering of abandoned projects and ideas is like the graveyard. It holds so much unrealized potential that got buried.

Do you want to continue on this path of uncertainty? For example, do you struggle to design your diet according to your gym routine in order to get the most desirable results? Let me guess: you started out strong for the first couple of weeks. You meal-prepped your food the night before your workout. You created a nutritional system to let you know how much protein, carbohydrates, and healthy fats to consume for each meal. Then, for no apparent reason, you just stopped and drifted back to your old haphazard pattern, consuming anything that delighted your taste buds.

Perhaps you managed to design a workout plan for yourself. You got tired of being a scatterbrain and formulated a plan that would allow you to exercise and hit every body part within a week. You were no longer going to work on your favorite machines randomly. You got into the groove and started to see results because not one muscle group was missed. But suddenly, in the blink of an eye, you found yourself exercising only chest and arms or just hitting the elliptical for the entire week.

Or you plan to go to the gym more frequently with an accountability partner to assist you. At this point, things are going well. You are encouraged by having a buddy by your side, striving for the same goal. Competition fuels the two of you, causing both of you to work harder to reach your goals faster. But the unexpected happens: your gym partner starts to become too busy to go to the gym with you. Excuses start creeping out of the woodwork. One week, it's "I'm sick." The next week, it's "I have so much to do." And the following week, he or she has to bathe the dog. Now you're no longer going to the gym either. You're back to square one.

Sound familiar? The same routine of starting something and not following through? Have you ever wondered why this is a pattern in almost everything you do? Well, let's look at possible underlying causes. What emotion triggered you to start eating better for your workout and caused you to meal-prep your food? Were you frightened by a story you read about a person who was diagnosed with morbid obesity and struggled through life with medical complications? Again, what emotion stirred you to create a weekly exercise plan for your entire body? Were you envious at the sight of a guy with six-pack abs on the beach or the woman with an hourglass figure? What emotion caused you to find an accountability partner for the gym? Was it a sense of insecurity? Did you feel you needed the support of a friend to help you along the way? Didn't you trust yourself enough to be accountable to yourself?

Recognize that these strong emotions that spurred you to embark on great things were only momentary and consequently developed to only temporary habits. These habits would last you only a couple of weeks before you crashed and slid into your old ways again. The lesson is to be wary of the emotions that drive you to do things for momentary gain and to never allow these emotions to control you. Be moved by your stronger convictions.

Increasing Willpower

To be consistent in an inconsistent world, the primary thing is to increase your willpower. What is willpower?

- The ability to delay gratification, resisting short-term temptations in order to meet long-term goals[6]
- The capacity to override an unwanted thought, feeling, or impulse
- Conscious, disciplined regulation of the self by the self

If you want to develop a willpower of steel aligned with your goals, you have three foundations to build on: motivation, detailed goal-setting, and self-control. Before I get into these three components, I want to address the notion that willpower is a limited resource. Over the last several years, numerous case studies illustrated that willpower is a discipline that can be depleted over time. Do I agree with this view? Yes and no. I agree because, if someone is trying to reach a particular goal, and they are going through tremendous obstacles over a long timeframe without seeing tangible progress, then the person may lose faith. As a result, their willpower can be depleted and they will never reach their goal. However, I strongly believe that most human attributes such as willpower will erode if operated under our own strength. Let me explain. If we start to increase our faith and place our strength in a higher source, a higher power like God, our willpower will never be depleted because we are receiving our power from an unlimited source. This principle is based on faith and will take time to master-I just wanted to share my views here. But for now, let's go back to the discussion of motivation, detailed goal-setting, and self-control.

MOTIVATION
Let's see if we can incorporate the concept of willpower in the first scenario just described. In the scenario of creating a nutritional plan for eating strategically to reach your fitness goal, your strong willpower makes you picture the body of your dreams taking shape. This desirable outcome motivates you to eat efficiently.

DETAILED GOAL-SETTING
Next, your goal has to be detail oriented so that you can focus on executing the blueprint of the eating plan you

formulated. If your eating plan is designed to lose body fat and gain lean muscle, you would need a high-protein, low-carbohydrate diet and a moderate intake of healthy fats.

In contrast, if your goal is to bulk up and gain muscle mass, you must have a high protein and carbohydrate intake with a moderate level of healthy fats. You also need to see that your calorie intake increases beyond your normal baseline. Lastly, you must exert the willpower to stay on track and not give in to the smallest temptations, such as chocolate cake, as opposed to an apple. And as you are in the process of bulking up, you must have the self-control to increase your caloric intake to gain the added mass.

SELF-CONTROL

Third, you need to consciously exercise self-control. In the case of the gym partner, because you needed a partner to keep up the momentum, you made the false assumption that you couldn't do it on your own. You became dependent on your partner. Consider how capable you were in motivating someone to exercise with you. Now use that same confidence to double-push yourself. To detail-orientate this goal, you must first address the possibility of what could go wrong to affect your outcome. In this case, there was a high probability that your gym partner could bail out. Your detail-oriented goal should therefore be to consistently go to the gym even if your partner doesn't show up.

The importance of self-control in the above scenario cannot be overstated. You must have the self-control not to allow your gym partner to disrupt the pattern of consistency you are building. In other words, tell yourself you may have to work out alone sometimes and have the self-control to push through. The detailed-oriented approach will make you accountable to each fitness milestone and will help you take ownership of it as your own.

Use the above three foundations of motivation, detailed goal-setting, and self-control to formulate a workout regimen that allows you to work on particular body parts rather than exercising aimlessly without a plan. You'll have to stay motivated and create a realistic program that targets your entire body. The detail-oriented goals should aim to work out every body part with the same effort and should not focus on just the body part you prefer. Self-control should constrain you from working out a certain body part more strenuously than the others, unless you have an asymmetrical figure with a heavy upper body but skinny legs or great tone everywhere except for a pudgy gut.

Building Consistency and Willpower

I recommend five methods you could implement on a daily basis that would help you to increase your consistency and willpower:

- Forming macro and micro habits
- Creating the "If…then" statement for each new habit
- Limiting your options in order to concentrate on the new habit
- Visualizing the new habit
- Protecting "your baby" from failing

FORMING MACRO AND MICRO HABITS

A macro habit relates to the big goal you would like to accomplish. Let's say your goal is to run a total of 155 miles in a month. To do so, you will first have to figure out the micro goals, or milestones, that would help you achieve your macro goal. So you decide to run five miles on the first of the month. You then calculate that you must run five miles each day of the month to reach 155 miles before the end of the month.

Using the macro and micro habit technique would put you on track. It allows you to work on the smaller milestones on a daily basis so that you can see intermediate successes on the way to your long-term goal. These achievements will allay anxiety and suppress the tendency to overload yourself in your enthusiasm to reach your target faster.

CREATING THE "IF…THEN" STATEMENT

Let's take running the 155 miles. Instead of saying that you have to run 155 miles before the month is over, use the

"If…then" technique to rephrase it as follows: **if** I run only five miles a day for the next thirty-one days, **then** I would be able to complete 155 miles for the month. Do you see the difference? The first statement tends to overwhelm because of the magnitude of the task. But the second statement breaks down the same goal into realistic mini goals and appears more doable and easier to accomplish.

Limiting Your Options

Having multiple goals within the same time frame may not be a wise move. The fewer goals you choose, the easier it is to concentrate on accomplishing them. The more goals you have running parallel, the less likely your chances are of fulfilling all of them. All of your efforts at consistency and hard work would go to waste. Ideally, you should focus on just one goal at a time to maximize your chances of reaching it and establishing the new habit of consistency.

Visualizing Your New Habit

Create a mental picture of yourself running every day till you finally celebrate the completion of your 155-mile target for the month. Without visualization, your new habit would be too remote and difficult to get excited about. It's like wanting to own a brand-new Mercedes but never dreaming of sitting in one, smelling the fresh leather interior, and hearing the purr of the engine as you turn on the ignition.

Protecting Your Baby

What do I mean by "your baby"? It's your fragile, newly birthed habit. New habits are prone to be discarded if they are not jealously protected. With any negative thought, the influence of others or life's ups and downs could easily eat away at your new habit of consistency, the motivation to attain a goal, your willpower, and, ultimately, your pursuit of grit. So reinforce your new habit of consistency with renewed motivation, self-control, and determination.

Mind-Body Medicine

You can use additional techniques to train your mind to be more consistent and honed to a higher level than where your natural impulses would lead you. This technique is mind-body medicine.[7] Mind-body medicine uses the power of thought and emotion to influence physical health. It trains the mind to focus solely on the body's wellbeing. You could use a number of techniques under mind-body medicine to enable you to be more consistent and stronger willed, but the two I want to introduce to you are *biofeedback* and *relaxation techniques*.

Biofeedback

Biofeedback enables you to control your involuntary bodily functions, such as your heart rate and blood pressure, to name a few. A technician attaches a device to you to monitor your internal functionality feedback. This would help you to observe your feedback so that you could mentally control it.

An example of the biofeedback technique would be the following:

- Let's say you want to undergo a stress test because your personal issues are pulling you down. The stress-test meter would indicate you are stressed, and if so, the technician would ask you to reminisce about a time when you were happiest. You start thinking about your great-grandmother and how she used to make homemade biscuits and jelly on Saturday morning in her house down an unpaved road in South Carolina. The meter starts to change momentarily, indicating a decrease of stress simply because of the alteration of your thought.

Relaxation Techniques

Relaxation techniques also help keep the mind calm despite the downward thrust of strong negative emotions. Now the mind can be completely focused on the body without any interruption.

Here is one relaxation technique I would highly recommend:

- If you struggle with depression and anxiety, the spiritual dimension of relaxation would definitely help. People diagnosed with depression or anxiety generally feel they are going through life isolated and alone. But through spiritual consciousness, they realize they always have a loving Father they can turn to. Studies have shown that AIDS patients who had a strong belief system, faith in a higher power, and a positive disposition accompanied by a caring attitude for others experienced a longer life expectancy than AIDS patients who did not practice any form of spirituality.[7]

How did I deal with developing the consistency habit? I confess that consistency was an ongoing issue for me. I would regularly go to the gym three days a week but would prefer to go six. Sometimes, due to lack of organization, I would not have eaten sufficiently throughout the day to sustain me for my workout. This would, of course, affect my performance. My workout plan also was unorganized. I did not conscientiously create an exercise plan for each week. Instead I made a mental note and worked out the muscles I did not focus on the previous day so that I could target a different body part.

I blamed such inconsistency on my ADHD, which makes me tend to focus on a single task and neglect other peripheral areas. This habit started during my college days.

In Pursuit of Grit

Because I was not consistent in studying for my exams, I would be in the library from dawn to dusk, cramming for an exam at the last minute, and I would not eat for the entire day until I had finished studying.

On the other hand, what really worked for me the most were the macro and micro habits and praying to God. Since my attention span is limited, I can assimilate this method because the tasks are broken down into smaller pieces that add up to the completion of my goal. The technique helped me to be more consistent than ever. It minimized procrastination and suppressed my natural wiring to start a task and not finish it. I realized that praying to God was extremely vital in making my weaknesses my strengths. Whenever I felt depleted in my own strength, I would pray to God and hand over my weaknesses to Him in faith, hoping He would convert them into my strengths. Miraculously, my prayers were answered every time.

I must confess that ADHD really had my goals and desires at a standstill at one point. I would see dramatic improvements in the strength of my willpower alone and my grades on my exams. But after a while, my body development would reach a plateau, and my grades would drop way below the potential I knew I had.

That said, I am grateful to have the benefit of research, medical assistance, and support systems to be better equipped to deal with my condition. Above all, it was practicing the techniques I discovered to combat ADHD—pursuing grit and striving to be the optimal version of myself—that have paid off immeasurably.

On the third and fourth weeks, use the combination of self-affirmation and techniques to strengthen the power of the mind to construct the foundation of acquiring a new habit.

Three

The Pleasure Principle versus the Reality Principle: The My-Body-Is-Too-Sore Excuse

And perseverance, character;
and character, hope.

—Romans 5:4

After a long break, you're finally back in the gym. This time, you are extremely focused. Your diet has been exactly right for the strenuous workout session. Your mind is ready to push it to no limit. You are adding heavier weights than usual. The reps for each exercise are through the roof. Your endurance seems stronger than ever. Sweat is dripping off you as though someone threw a bucket of water in your face. You are striving through the pain as the lactic acid is building up in your muscles. You are lifting fifty-pound dumbbells at an incline chest press for muscle mass. You're performing twenty-five repetitions of squats for definition in one sitting. You've been burning fat while on the step master for an hour and a half.

For the first time in a long while, you impress yourself. As your session comes to a close, you can barely walk. The particular body part you worked on is sore. You are breathing heavily, and your heart is beating at an astronomical rate, to the point where you can hear it in your head. As you are approaching the exit, you are so amped about today's performance. You cannot wait for tomorrow to do it again.

The following morning, on the verge of waking up, you discover that getting out of bed is a challenge because of the soreness from yesterday's epic workout. So you give yourself a reward and decide not to go to the gym.

Yesterday's workout was the best performance ever. You can't dispute that. But what went wrong? You are sore. So how about your workout today? Are you going to let the pain stop you? How do you expect to lose the weight? Can you imagine taking a day or two off every time you're sore? With that pattern, you'll never have the body you dream of or reach your personal fitness goals. Are you going to let pain stop your progress?

Have you heard of the butterfly story? The story is about a young biology student who felt sorry to see a pupa struggling to get out of its chrysalis. He decided to give the pupa a hand by carefully making an incision along its chrysalis and easing it out slowly. A beautiful butterfly emerged. Unfortunately, the butterfly could not fly because its wings were not fully formed. It needed the struggle out of the chrysalis to develop the strength to have the ability to fly.

They say you could always learn a lesson from small creatures like insects. The lesson is that struggle and pain are necessary for mental and physical growth. You have to experience some sort of struggle or pain in life or else you would be handicapped and unable to get out of a tough situation. The fact is this: pain is essential to the development of character and growth. You can't live your life without pain because it instills vital survival tools—character building, perseverance, and growth, to name a few. If you try dodging any encounter with pain, you will not experience life to the fullest. You will never be challenged and will therefore never experience victory.

Once pain starts to knock on your door and you don't let it in, another character, ease, will invade your home and rob you of your prized possessions, your dreams, and your time. Instead, brace yourself for pain's visit and offer it a cup of coffee once it knocks; don't ignore it.

I mentioned two new concepts—self-affirmation and the power of the mind—in the previous two chapters. I am now going to let you in on a third secret of how to improve your grit for your workout and for your life. It's the tussle between the pleasure principle and the reality principle. Let me take a moment to explain how both principles operate in psychological terms.

The Id, Ego, and Superego[8]

The renowned psychoanalyst Sigmund Freud identified three driving forces in the human personality: the id, the ego, and the superego. The id is the part we know from birth. It's the most primal part of us. It operates by instinct according to the pleasure principle and demands satisfaction every time there is a need or want. A baby, for instance, feels hungry and demands milk. If it is denied its milk, it throws a tantrum. The pleasure principle therefore expects immediate gratification or fulfillment of its wants and desires.

The next driver of personality is the ego, or self-concept. As we mature, we become conscious of our need for acceptance and recognition in society. We adopt socially acceptable behavior because we realize that rules and regulations are necessary in a civilized society. We therefore learn to modify our behavior according to the reality principle. The reality principle teaches us to control our basic emotions and behave in a civilized way.

For example, you are thirsty as you drive along the highway and long for a beer. But you can control this desire, knowing that the driving-while-intoxicated law makes it illegal to drink alcohol while driving, so you wait until you get home. The pleasure principle is now bowing to the reality principle through a process known as "deferred gratification." The ego also drives us to achieve our ambitions, improve our station in life, and pursue other higher goals.

The highest driver of personality is the superego. This aspect of our personality causes us to develop moral judgments and loftier aspirations, such as compassion for the handicapped and seeking the good of the community. Our superego enables us to rise above our primal instincts to strive for goals larger than our personal desires. It teaches us to make sacrifices for the sake of others.

In fact, our adult life is a constant tussle between the id demanding immediate attention according to the pleasure principle and the ego and superego constraining us by the reality principle. By applying the reality principle, we learn to defer gratification and to pursue loftier goals. The more we operate by the reality principle in pursuit of grit, the more we can develop our self-control and willpower to override our basic instincts.

With the reality principle now established in your mind, even as pain inflicts your body, you intentionally reorientate it to view things in a different perspective. When you wake up with your quads swelling or your bicep sore as it protrudes out of your sleeve, or you begin to notice a couple of inches off your waistline, tell yourself that's a sign of growth and change. You are meeting your objectives. You finally conclude that pain is necessary for your development, not just for the gym but outside the gym as well. You begin to look at your pain as a positive indicator of something good happening rather than as a negative experience.

So on your way back to the gym, sore from your previous workout, tell yourself, "This is a good kind of pain." Your body will slowly become less conscious of the soreness and start to respond differently to that pain. If you don't learn to welcome the pain, to endure it, and to start appreciating the discomfort (as an indicator of ultimate success), you will never see progress in your discipline, willpower, or development of grit.

In Pursuit of Grit

Imbued with the reality principle, your mind will allow itself to be constantly exposed to pain because it subconsciously recognizes the pain as a gateway to ultimate victory. And in return, your body will desire to work out despite the pain. Eventually, with the assimilation of the reality principle, your mind and body will adapt to the exposure of pain during and after a workout to the point that both develop an appreciation for the pain. They will eventually reject the id's tendency to flee from pain at all costs.

As a person with ADHD, I am well aware that I am programmed to operate more by the pleasure principle than the reality principle.[9] People with ADHD have a disorder in the brain because the gray matter is noticeably smaller than that of normal people. This gray matter serves as an information processor that controls neuron and communication functions. This definitely explains the struggles I had with poor communication skills for many years.

People who suffer from ADHD are also very impulsive. The id component of our personality is the driving force. My impulsiveness is more pronounced in my communication with people. I would usually talk without thinking of the repercussions. Some people refer to this as has having "no filter."

Let me show you the effect of ADHD on my brain and how I used to operate in the id. Let's say it's a snowy day, and my wife puts on her high heels, knowing there is a pair of boots in the car. I tell her she should put on her sneakers, but she's already out of the house and wearing the high heels. Seconds later, she slips and falls. The right response should be, "Are you okay, honey?"

But it's not. Since ADHD takes off the filters, my first reaction is, "I told you not to wear the high heels and to put on the sneakers!" Only after that would I ask, "Are you okay, honey?"

My wife would then look at me as if I were a totally insensitive brute. But my heart's intention was to show concern.

Or perhaps because of my id-driven behavior, I recklessly go to the gym and pick up the heaviest weight, hoping to accelerate my body development. Keep in mind that I am also operating in my strong willpower, so I have no doubt at all that the weight could be lifted. But is it wise? No, it's not. That's why I have to train myself to operate more in the reality principle. But my disorder tugs at me not to do so because it prefers the pleasure principle. Aha! That's where the pursuit of grit comes in for me. Uncomfortable or not, I have to go against my mental bent and follow the reality principle.

All in all, it's been a lot of work, but it's paying off. In the pursuit of grit, I have been able to alter my brain functionality when I've submitted to various treatments, such as going to the gym more frequently, increasing my organization skills, setting realistic goals for myself, and creating a daily routine and sticking to it.

I am happy to report that these treatments have brought about the following benefits:

- Improvement in performance at the gym and in everyday tasks
- Reduced occurrence of starting a task and not finishing it
- Progress toward the goals I strongly desire
- Improvement in social and communication skills

Higher-Level Goals

To really grasp the reality principle, we have to tune the mind to aim for higher-level goals. Far-reaching goals give the most satisfying rewards. However, these higher long-term goals demand perseverance, sacrifice, discomfort, and often pain.

I will illustrate this concept using three typical real-life scenarios that must operate under the reality principle and that would crumble under the pleasure principle. These scenarios are *getting out of debt, starting a profitable business,* and *getting a college degree while working a nine-to-five job.*

GETTING OUT OF DEBT

In the process of getting out of debt, you must first have the patience, self-control, and determination to eventually pay back everyone you owe. Your patience controls the desire to operate in the pleasure principle and expect your appetites to be satisfied. Of course you desire to pay off your debts all at once, but you have to manage your limited resources. Self-control is vital to managing your cash flow. It helps you live within your budget and avoid frivolous spending, such as spending ten dollars a day to buy lunch instead of bringing home-cooked lunches to work. The determination to put things in perspective will enable you to understand why you must deny your immediate desires to achieve the goal of being debt-free.

STARTING A PROFITABLE BUSINESS

The reality principle must definitely govern starting a profitable business. You cannot cut corners when it comes to starting a business venture. The discomfort may be the risk of investing your hard-earned money in a business that may or may not turn out to be profitable. You would also have to sacrifice a tremendous amount of time and effort to get it off the ground for the first couple of years.

In Pursuit of Grit

Immediate gratification rarely occurs in a new business, so you are already primed to operate under the reality principle and prepared to make sacrifices for long-term gains. If a business operates under the pleasure principle, such as overpricing goods and services in unreasonable ways for the customer, then the business would quickly fail.

GETTING A COLLEGE DEGREE

Now, this scenario is difficult: working a full-time job while trying to acquire a college degree at the same time. Many people have done this, including myself. I remember going to college to pursue a degree in health information technology and simultaneously working a forty-hour week at a retail store. This wasn't easy. I had to make sure my grades were good enough to graduate while I also performed well at my job to maintain my expenses and funding for textbooks, tuition, and so on. Juggling the two was truly challenging because my ADHD complicated any attempt at multitasking. But I had set my sights on my college degree with the greater long-term assurance of gainful employment.

If I had operated in the pleasure principle, while maintaining my job and pursuing a higher education, I would have lost my job due to poor attendance and tardiness. It is also likely I would not have attained my college degree because I would not have studied. I know without a doubt, if I had falling prey to the pleasure principle, it would have cost me my job or my degree and that would have affected my future to the point that this book would not even have been conceived.

In conclusion, for you to achieve success in your personal development, at the gym, and in anything you do in life, the reality principle has to guide you. Could you imagine operating under the pleasure principle and demanding that your primal impulses be satisfied all the time? You would never get anywhere, and your world would be totally chaotic and uncivilized.

During the fifth and sixth weeks, accumulate and implement all the strategies that you learned to continue transforming your bad habits into new, positive ones with self-affirmations, the power of the mind, and the reality principle versus the pleasure principle. At this point, you are three-fifths on the verge of creating new habits that will alter your life.

Four

THE VISIONARY'S RECONSTRUCTION:
THE SEE-NO-RESULTS EXCUSE

In order to carry a positive action, we
must develop here a positive vision.

—DALAI LAMA

The gym has been your sanctuary from the outside world. You can release stress and finally focus on the one who's been neglected and who matters most: you. You're the healthiest you've ever been in years. Your dietary consumption is astonishing. You've discarded all artificial sugars from your eating regime, you're indulging in the finest non-GMO organic foods and vegetables, and you're eating lean meats from your local farms and wild-caught fish.

There's just one problem: you are not seeing any immediate results. The frustration is unbearable. You start questioning whether you are really spending your time well, wondering if all the effort has gone to nothing. You breathe in, studying yourself in the mirror a dozen times a day, but you don't see any changes in your physique. In your mind, the walls are closing in, and it's time to get off this path. It's true that you have disciplined yourself for so long, but now a sense of futility in going through the same regimen is creeping in. Countless hours of prepping meals and going to the gym in all weather conditions may have been an unnecessary punishment. With a helpless sigh, you throw in the towel and stop going to the gym entirely.

So after weeks of working out, you've decided to give up the gym because you weigh the same and the flab is still showing. Why throw away all the hard work so easily? Don't you value the precious time you've invested in yourself? Also, keep in mind that your eyes can play tricks. For the greater part of the time, you are not likely to see any dramatic change in your appearance. It will often take someone else to notice the sudden change you've worked so hard for.

It's worth mentioning that you may not see the weight loss because you've shed inches as opposed to pounds. You may not notice the muscle mass, but I can guarantee that you are getting stronger. A champion doesn't quit, regardless of how difficult it is to attain his or her goal. You know you're a true champion, right? As a champion, you already know that success doesn't come easy. It takes perseverance and dedication in your journey to victory.

Let me take this time to remind you that a champion is not someone who has never been defeated but is someone who experiences defeat after defeat but gets back up to walk the road to glory. *Failure* has been deleted from your vocabulary.

In the past chapters, we talked about self-affirmation, the power of the mind, and the pleasure principle versus the reality principle, three of the five secrets to strengthen your grit. I am now going to unleash the fourth secret: the visionary's reconstruction. The basis of this principle is that your vision primarily drives your emotions. Therefore, the vision of a desirable outcome that will embed positive emotions in your subconscious should always accompany your positive self-affirmations. Positive visuals are a wellspring of life: they bring encouragement, hope, and affirmation. Positive visions revive ambition. On the other hand, emotions like fear and doubt are rooted in the visions of defeat and failure that negative thoughts trigger.

You must now reconstruct your vision and self-image by using words that produce the most desirable emotions for optimal results. In this case, where you avoided going to the gym because you didn't see any results, images associated with "failure" shrouded your vision, and your vision was conceived in defeat. Reconstruction must take place to repair the damage done. Practice the habit of reprogramming your vision, and rise from the abyss of failure, which produces mediocrity, to the heights of greatness, which produce victory.

If you feel like you are not seeing results in the gym, start to change your perception of yourself. See yourself as a winner. See the end results, not the setbacks. Continue to eat right and be consistent in your workout regimen. Continue to declare these self-affirmations:

- "I will lose the weight."
- "I will acquire the muscle mass."
- "I will be toned."

While you are saying these self-affirmations, attach a vision for each:

- "I will lose the weight."—"I can see myself losing twenty pounds."
- "I will acquire the muscle mass."—"I see myself already having the muscle mass."
- "I will be toned."—"Being jacked is not an option; it's already done."

This reconstruction of your visuals is crucial, especially when there are roadblocks in the process of reaching your goals. Reconstruction provides your willpower with all the necessary emotional support to break through all barriers and be reenergized for your task.

Ways to Optimize Your Visualization

You could use various techniques to enhance your visualization. Consider the mental image you want to display in your mind to help you execute a desirable outcome. For example, imagine yourself running a marathon or looking proudly at your well-defined physique. Playing that imagery over and over again is the key. Here are four ways to optimize your powers of visualization:

Method One: Design a Creative Atmosphere

To let your visualization flourish, think about redesigning your environment to stimulate your five senses to produce the mood you desire. Different atmospheres appeal to different people. Some people need upbeat music to stimulate their creativity. For others, it's natural sounds, such as the patter of rain or the birds chirping. Others function best in complete silence. The atmosphere in your working environment is also important for fresh ideas to spring forth. Could it be a walk in the

park or a drive in the countryside? Or sitting in a bou-
levard café while enjoying the aroma of freshly brewed
coffee?

If you are one of those who do your best thinking in the
privacy of your study, have you thought about repainting
your walls? The colors you frequently surround yourself
with could alter your mood and emotions. The color yel-
low, for instance, is a warm color that generates energy,
while green promotes relaxation. The right ambience can
invigorate, soothe, or inspire, depending on the mood
that's called for.

Method Two: Learn Breathing Techniques

Breathing exercises are a great way to calm yourself if you
are overwhelmed or mentally scattered. Inhaling deeply
and prolonging your slow exhale sharpens your focus
and puts you in the right frame of mind to visualize. For
me, breathing exercises often produce an image of the
steadily-rippling waters of the ocean. That's how calm
and focused I am once I practice my breathing and peace
floods my soul.

Method Three: Visualize Your Achievements

Always dream big dreams, and visualize these achievements in the most vivid way possible so that they are
almost tangible. Try to engage all of your five senses to

make your vision multidimensional. If you are running a twenty-six mile marathon, smell the sweat of your hard work, feel the steady thud of your shoes hitting the track and the wind as you streak by your opponents, see the finish line, and hear the blare of loudspeakers proclaiming you the winner.

METHOD FOUR: ATTACH POSITIVE EMOTIONS TO EACH DREAM

This follows the law of attachment and might be the most vital method of them all. For each dream or vision you want to achieve, attach positive emotions to provide a compelling motivation.

In the above example of the marathon, engage your emotions to enjoy the sweat of your hard work, the zest of slicing through the wind, the thrill of overtaking your opponents, and the absolute euphoria of breaking through the finish line. Feel your heart swell with pride as the crowd thunders in applause. Keep replaying that scene.

Visualization has played a huge part in my achievement of personal goals. I came to realize there had to be a connection between the disparate experiences of discomfort, pain, willpower, and the pursuit of grit. Visualization became my chief method of connection. The strong imagery and positive emotions associated with visualization have produced a dynamic that works for good in the overall scheme of things.

Happily, ADHD did not affect me visually because I am a visual learner. Whatever my goals are, I have to imagine myself already accomplishing them. I always create mental pictures when it comes to reaching a goal I deeply desire. In the past, I would constantly replay my setbacks and other negative images of myself. However, during my training, I realized that all this negative imagery produced nothing but futility and defeat. I have since learned to replace regret for things done badly with optimism in every learning experience.

I personally use self-affirmation and visualization to assist me in the process of completing a task from start to finish. I could be performing in the gym or completing the writing of this very book, and I continue to create the right imagery to spur me on. The moment I stop, my dreams could very well be that—just dreams!

The seventh and eight weeks are crucial. You want to stay focused because you are approaching the sixty-six day that is known to be a plateau for many people and, as a result, discourages the continuation of the newly created habits. So, on that note, continue to be strong and to apply self-affirmation, the power of the mind, the reality principle versus the pleasure principle, and the visionary's reconstruction techniques. You are just days closer to attaining the new habits necessary for becoming your optimal self.

Five

The Mind's Comfort Zone: The Fear Excuse

The fear of man brings a snare.

—Proverbs 29:25

It's New Year's Day, the beginning of starting everything afresh. You decide to make a strict resolution for yourself: eliminate alcoholic beverages, refrain from eating out, concentrate on your health, and go to the gym. To start on your renewed mission, you go to the supermarket to purchase healthy food, and you rush to the athletic stores to buy a few workout outfits. You are all pumped up to begin the New Year on a good note.

Later in the day, you decide to go to the gym. Before going, you took a nice hot shower and put on one of the new gym outfits you just bought. As you approach the gym, through the window you can see a mass of people working out. It looks like a human stampede. After all the work you put into preparing yourself for this point, you decide to turn back home because you simply refuse to work out in a crowded gym.

Now, my question to you is this: Why does a crowded gym stop you in your tracks? Aren't you comfortable with having people around as you perform a squat? Do you suffer from agoraphobia? Do you consistently let other people be a potential obstacle in your life? If so, who's really in control of your destiny, you or others?

Consider this: If you had to go to the emergency room, would you decide to leave the hospital because you notice the waiting room is teeming with patients? When going to the gym, are you there for yourself or others? I can completely understand your fear if a crowded place is your phobia, but you still have to acknowledge your fear and confront it.

Maybe you were one of those students in third grade who was constantly teased because of your weight, and the harsh remarks made you self-conscious about your appearance. But if this is the case, are you going to allow the past to affect your adulthood? This fear of people's perceptions of you could easily consume you and hold you back when it comes to stepping out. I can empathize with your fear and the root of it because I've been there too. So my challenge to us is this: How are we going to convert this fear into strength? If we don't face it, it's always going to knock on our door for the rest of our lives until we finally answer it and face it head on.

You probably were once on a high school or college team, and you caught your breath when a counterpart's performance—especially if that counterpart was of the opposite sex—surpassed yours to the point that you had to retreat to the sidelines for a drink of water. Are you concerned that this blot on your record would transfer to your present performance in the gym and that everyone would see the opposite sex outdoing you?

Perhaps you were that awkward kid with antisocial tendencies in the back of the classroom, looking on as the cool kids received all the attention you secretly desired. This past experience could be suppressing your enjoyment of the gym. You would like to make small talk with the guys and gals in the room, but you feel you are just too socially awkward for any type of interaction. You just do your workout and leave unfulfilled because of the lack of human engagement. This state of fear is doing more harm than good. How would you know how to engage in communication if you don't try? You just have to do it. You might be missing out on a potential gym partner or, better yet, a friend.

Right now, think about five things you are not comfortable doing but know, deep within, that you have to do them. How would your life play out if you avoid the things you need to do because you're not comfortable doing them? Would you be living to your fullest potential if you backed away from everything that freaked you out? Would you be able to face the person looking back at you in the mirror, knowing you haven't challenged yourself to venture into new territory? Would you submit to failure simply because you haven't tried your very best?

Finally, we come to the last and ultimate step in the process of strengthening your willpower and pursuing grit for your workout and life's achievements. You already know about self-affirmation, the power of the mind, the pleasure principle versus the reality principle, and the visionary's reconstruction. I now welcome you to the last secret of your journey: the mind's comfort zone.

The mind's comfort zone is a comfortable and habitual place where your mind retreats to because it is conditioned to do so. It rejects or avoids unfamiliar situations, which it largely sees as a threat. You know the comfort zone can rob you of new opportunities and vistas, but you just feel uncomfortable stepping out. The key is to expand your comfort zone by making comfortable what the mind sees as uncomfortable. Using self-affirmation, you need to remind yourself that, whatever your discomfort is, you have to see and declare out loud what is now your comfort.

Some scientific techniques could assist you in facing and conquering your phobia of the unfamiliar. One technique that could help you is called cognitive behavior therapy (CBT), also known as behavioral therapy or psychotherapy.[10] CBT is psychotherapy that combines cognitive therapy with behavior therapy. In other words, it merges understanding the root of a problem with modifying your behavior to correct it. CBT identifies faulty or dysfunctional patterns of thinking, feeling, or behaving and substitutes them with wholesome thoughts, healthy emotional responses, and socially acceptable behavior.

In addition, to help you venture beyond the mind's comfort zone, I would like to introduce the process of exposure therapy. Exposure therapy is essential to expanding the mind's comfort zone because it allows an unfamiliar situation or scenario to be transformed into a nonthreatening ground for you to extend your comfort zone to. This inevitably makes the potential threat a safe place.

A good example of this is when your phobia is the fear of heights, but you challenge yourself to face it directly by getting on a roller coaster at a theme park and having the time of your life.[11] Exposure therapy modifies the irrational fear associated with a situation by first activating the fear and then providing new information to downgrade the fear or unrealistic associations. For example, we can speak to ourselves calmly and rationally that tachycardia does not lead to heart attacks. Neither do crowded malls lead to terrorist attacks. By the conscious act of confronting the feared stimulus or responses and adding corrective information to our fear bank, we can gradually cause the fear to subside.

What causes you to panic or be fearful? Snakes? Spiders? Driving? Flying? Sleeping in strange places? For many people, it's the fear of public speaking. The underlying principle to overcome the fear is to first get your rational mind to recognize that a large part of the fear is self-induced and irrational. The next step is to expose you to the specific fearful experience in a controlled setting where the risk is minimized. People who are terrified of public speaking first learn to interact with other learners in small buzz groups where they receive affirmation and encouragement. Once their confidence is built up, they start addressing a supportive audience.

Let me ask you a question: Could a strainer contain the substance of water? The answer is both yes and no. No, because water in its natural state would go right through the strainer. But if the water molecules were modified and became frozen, then they could be retained. In the same way, pretend you are the water and the strainer is your fear. If you allow your fears to consume you, you would be like the natural state of water and lose yourself through the strainer.

But if you alter the way you think, just as the water molecules altered themselves into solid form, then you would stand solid amid the fearful situation. You would not allow fear to control you or change or distort your perceptions. Your thinking would align with the objective facts and disassociate from those that your imagination or bad memories have colored. You would be able to rightly assess the risks at hand and recognize those that have been irrationally magnified through your own negative experiences. Once you can clearly see who is in control, you can climb out of the strainer you were poured into like water and stand on solid ground, free of your phobias.

Now let's play back the scene where you were looking through the window of the gym. Now that you have the concept of the mind's comfort zone firmly planted within you, you are more equipped to make a better decision. As you observe the mass of people exercising through the fogged window, you step inside the gym, having taken a deep breath to calm your nerves. You approach the customer service counter to sign up for a one-year membership at the gym. Once you get your membership card, you walk toward the free weights in the middle of people exercising. Once you grab the twenty-pound dumbbell, you intentionally look into the mirror and say to yourself, "I am comfortable," and you start your workout with only you in mind.

As the session goes on, it's as if you're the only one in the gym. Your focus is tunnel vision. Your self-affirmation is on point, with no trace of negative, hindering words. You are impressing on your mind the desire to be in a crowded environment. You are slowly implementing the power of the mind. The words you are expelling under your breath, "I am comfortable," are slowly dispelling the unease of being in the presence of so many people. The reality principle has become your ally in this moment.

While your eyes are pierced to the ceiling of the gym as you perform an incline dumbbell fly, you can envision yourself going to the gym every time the gym is crowded, accompanied by words of encouragement. You have attached the last link to the chain of strong willpower with the combination of the visionary's reconstruction and altering the mind's comfort zone. You are on the brink of a purposeful future by applying the five secret strategies—self-affirmation, the power of the mind, the pleasure principle versus the reality principle, the visionary's reconstruction, and the mind's comfort zone—to possessing the character of grit.

I know personally how fears could have enslaved you in a prison within yourself. Do you want to continue to be a slave of your phobias, or do you want to break free of the bondages and start living your life? My secret fear has been claustrophobia. This stemmed from my childhood, where I remember my older siblings would bury me under a mountain of clothes and sit on top of it. I would scream at the top of my lungs but would only get relief moments later, not right away. For a young child, this was extremely traumatizing. This fear would grow and manifest itself into being afraid of elevators. Then it would expand to more closed-in environments, such as a closed MRI machine.

To be honest with you, I must have been trapped in an elevator so many times that it got to the point where I no longer was afraid, and I would just shrug my shoulders and say to myself in a nonchalant way, "Here we go again!" When I was trying to discover what was going on with me mentally, I was referred to a neurologist. After consultation, the neurologist scheduled an MRI on my brain. I vividly remember sitting in the waiting room, tensely anticipating this ordeal. There was a long wait for the open MRI machine, and the closed one was ironically available. I decided to undergo the procedure regardless.

Once inside the closed MRI, my heart started palpitating so hard that I could hear it thud. However, I concentrated on my breathing and said aloud to myself, "Don't be afraid. You're not going to die." I continued focusing on my breathing until the procedure was over. I would say it lasted fifteen to twenty minutes, but to someone overwhelmed by fear, it seemed like a lifetime.

One thing about me is that I try to face my phobias directly, so I am repeatedly performing self-exposure therapy on myself. The more I expose myself to my fears, the more my phobias become my strength. I am extremely proud of myself for facing my fears and continuing to do so. Self-exposure therapy is a great way to slowly chip away at your phobias. But again, it's your choice whether you want to be a prisoner within yourself or use the key to unlock endless possibilities.

Within the last three weeks of acquiring your new habits, which is the ninth through eleventh weeks, you are now equipped with a new, life-changing habit. You will start to see how each technique is slowly manifesting in every aspect of your life. The implementation of all five secret strategies—self-affirmations, the power of the mind, the reality principle versus the pleasure principle, the visionary's reconstruction, and the mind's comfort zone—is the ultimate guide in becoming the person you always desired.

The power you hold within your hand isn't just for inside the gym. It's also for outside—for life. These five secrets have now become your inner voice; these five vital gems are now integrated in your habitual behavior. Now you're officially ready to go on the hunt in pursuit of grit!

Six

The Road to Glory:
Victory at All Costs

*Victory at all costs, victory in spite of
all terror, victory however long and
hard the road may be; for without
victory, there is no survival.*

—Winston Churchill

I was approaching the office of my neuropsychologist
two weeks after taking an extensive eight-hour exam
to see what was wrong with me. I thought I already knew
the diagnosis. Yes, I had diagnosed myself and was totally
convinced I had dyslexia. But I was so wrong. My doctor, accompanied with a colleague, sat down with me and

said, "Darrell, you don't have dyslexia, but you do have attention deficit hyperactivity disorder." By way of consolation, he said it was better to have ADHD than dyslexia since there were more resources, treatments, and material on ADHD.

When that acronym was pronounced, I was at a loss for words. I said under my breath, "I feel so hopeless," but by the same token, I also felt a sense of relief. My doctor and his colleague assured me I shouldn't feel hopeless. They gave me a variety of suggestions to assist me in my treatment. They mentioned I had the option of taking prescription drugs to help combat ADHD and live a normal life. They also recommended purchasing three books: *The Memory Bible* by Gary Small, MD; *Your Memory* by Kenneth L. Higbee, PhD; and *Achieve Optimal Memory* by Aaron P. Nelson, PhD, with Susan Gilbert. Lastly, I was to make an appointment to see a therapist.

I decided to purchase the books first to know more about this diagnosis. I became fascinated with the medical journals on ADHD and the effects it had on every aspect of my life until all this information overwhelmed me. It was simply amazing to have had this disorder all my life and only now, at the age of thirty-four, discover it. No one—not my parents, siblings, close relatives, teachers, or coworkers—had a clue. No one, not even the closest one to me, myself.

I finally willed myself to stop being overwhelmed by all the information I was absorbing about the detrimental effects of ADHD on my mind. As I decided not to submit to but to grapple with the disorder, I suddenly had a mind shift. I could steady my mind to think calmly and rationally. Clarity and positive thinking began to form. I began to apply in my daily life much of the useful information I had obtained and even formulated my own strategies to reprogram everything that the disorderly filter of ADHD tainted. Much of my perception of the world and how I viewed myself and conversed with my loved ones, colleagues at work, strangers, and, most importantly, myself was wrong. I learned that to be able to learn about my true self, I had to focus on self-awareness.

I gradually started cultivating new habits through the techniques I had learned. To my delight, I found my self-talk and self-control improving, my willpower strengthening, my procrastination minimizing, my cognitive skills enhancing, and, most importantly, this thing called *grit* coming into sight.

The accumulation of these techniques I stumbled upon in my search for knowledge began to combine well with the methods I learned on my own to combat ADHD. I started to conscientiously apply these principles and, to my surprise, found they were really effective in my mental ability to fight against ADHD.

The practice of self-affirmation has helped me to develop an unbreakable self-concept system that no one on this green earth could take away. My confidence has soared to the skies. This concept has really helped me push through to complete a given task—of which the writing of this book is a sterling example.

I am also applying the power of the mind for optimal results. Harnessing the power of the mind has helped me realize that willpower is not a limited resource, according to popular belief, but an immeasurable resource with no limits if you are willing to take authority of your situation. Because ADHD feeds my habit of inconsistency, the power of the mind grabs ADHD by the horns and shows it who's boss.

The visionary's reconstruction is one of my favorite concepts. I have enhanced my ability to visualize what I want as a tangible thing to be captured in pursuit of an intangible goal. I might find myself in an unfavorable situation, but I keep my vision strong, reinforced by my positive motivation and stable emotions. I might not see the full result of my labor, yet I know it's near because my imagery is so close to reality.

In Pursuit of Grit

I would have to say the mind's comfort zone might be the second-most uncomfortable of all the concepts. But for some strange reason, I am in love with discomfort. Having the ability to stare fear dead in the eye is truly liberating. The ability to convert my phobias into potential strengths is an amazing breakthrough that definitely makes life worthwhile.

Finally, the reality principle versus the pleasure principle is the latest concept I discovered. This has actually been the most difficult for me to internalize, simply because my mind is designed to be id driven and impulsive, thanks to the hijacking nature of ADHD. According to a recent study, people diagnosed with ADHD are more likely to be involved in multiple car accidents. This is the drastic effect of impulsiveness that people like myself are plagued with on a daily basis. On that note, I have to be mindful of my impulsive ways since I am aware I need constant stimulation to be engaged, and often, impulsive urges or needs trigger my behavior. I am thankful I have gotten better at controlling these impulses, but it's going to take some time to master.

But the most valuable achievement, which I hold dear to my heart, is not any particular concept. It's my personal pursuit of grit. Through grit, I have been able to strengthen my character and become the man I've always wanted to be.

This journey of gathering and applying such vital information to anchor me could also be something that assists you! Yes, I am talking to *you*. Whatever your obstacles—inside or outside those gym doors—you now have the tools and the undergirding of grit to be victorious. This is your personal journey, but you definitely will not walk alone.

As you read this book and work on the solutions it prescribes for at least seventy-seven days, I will be by your side. Allow self-affirmations to be a part of your subconscious, make sacrifices to reach your long-term goals, engulf yourself in the sea of discomfort to grow in character and grit, change your perception and vision to see things in light instead of darkness, use willpower to break through internal and external obstacles, operate under the guidance of the reality principle to overcome instant gratification, and endure the pain that's necessary for your transformation. This is your certain way to victory. Allow your mind to be renewed according to all the concepts in this book, and you will experience your world opening up as you set yourself *in pursuit of grit*!

Definitions

The Power of the Mind is summoning your will to take control of your mind and make it desire what you desire it to do. This is where self-affirmation is vital because whatever your natural mind rejects through habit, your words will have to negate by declaring—out loud—positive outcomes. The idea is to train your mind into wanting what the natural mind would not have desired.

Self-Affirmation is the glue that binds each of the other four secrets. It enables you to say positive words to yourself out loud to strengthen your belief system and dismantle your self-doubt.

The Mind's Comfort Zone is when your natural mind has been conditioned to do things that are comfortable and performed in a habitual manner, but the key is to expand the mind's comfort zone by making what's uncomfortable for the natural mind comfortable for the renewed mind. With self-affirmation, you have to remind yourself that whatever is your "discomfort" is now your comfort. The process of exposure therapy is the main factor in reprogramming the mind's comfort zone. Exposure therapy is vital to the mind's comfort zone because it encourages you to confront your fears. It allows a situation that you are not familiar with—and therefore fearful of—to become a safe habitation. This inevitably makes your "discomfort" a comfort.

The Pleasure Principle is based on our primal instincts that developed from childhood. Its main purpose is to impulsively serve and fulfill its natural desires, and it operates by immediate gratification.

The Reality Principle helps us control our primal behavior and behave in a civilized way. The concept is to acquire deferred gratification in pursuit of long-term goals.

The Visionary's Reconstruction allows you to elicit the desired emotions to produce optimal results. Your words and visions drive your emotions. So your words of self-affirmation should always be positive, accompanied by a vision of a desirable outcome that will give rise to a positive emotion, such as encouragement and ambition. Opposed to this are emotions like fear and doubt, which are rooted in negative words and visions of defeat and failure.

Notes

Introduction

1. "Grit," *Merriam-Webster's Online Dictionary*, accessed March 21, 2017 https://www.merriam-webster.com/dictionary/grit

2. Lily Hechtman et al., "Treatment of Adults with Attention-Deficit/Hyperactivity Disorder, *Neuropsychiatry Disease and Treatment* 4, no. 2 (April 2008): 389–403, accessed March 21, 2017 https://www.ncbi.nlm.nih.gov/pmc/articles/PMC2518387/.

Chapter 1

3. A.M. Steinbach, "Neurolinguistic Programming: A Systematic Approach to Change," *Canadian Family Physician* 30 (January 1984):147–150, accessed March 21, 2017. https://www.ncbi.nlm.nih.gov/pmc/articles/PMC2153995/?page=1.

4. Ronald Alexander, "The Power of Affirmations: How to Make Them Work for You," October 9, 2011, *Huffington Post*, http://www.huffingtonpost.com/ronald-alexander-phd/positive-affirmations_b_921184.html. Accessed March 21, 2017.

5. Benjamin Gardner, "Making Health Habitual: The Psychology of 'Habit-Formation' and General Practice," *British Journal of General Practice* (December 2012): 664–666, https://www.ncbi.nlm.nih.gov/pmc/articles/PMC3505409/. Accessed March 21, 2017.

Chapter 2

6. Kirsten Weir, "What You Need to Know About Willpower: The Psychological Science of Self-Control," *APA.org*, last accessed, http://www.apa.org/helpcenter/willpower.aspx. Accessed March 21, 2017.

7. Steven D. Ehrlich, "Mind-Body Medicine," *University of Maryland Medical Center Medical Reference Guide*, last accessed, http://umm.edu/health/medical/altmed/treatment/mindbody-medicine. Accessed March 21, 2017.

Chapter 3

8. Kendra Cherry, "Psychology—What Are the Id, Ego, and Superego? The Structural Model of Personality," *Very Well*, last accessed, https://www.verywell.com/the-id-ego-and-superego-2795951. March 21, 2017.

9. Larry J. Seidman et al., "Gray Matter Alterations in Adults with Attention-Deficit/Hyperactivity Disorder

Identified by Voxel-Based Morphometry," *Biological Psychiatry* 69, no. 9 (May 1, 2011): 857–866, https://www.ncbi.nlm.nih.gov/pmc/articles/PMC3940267/. Accessed March 21, 2017.

Chapter 5

10. "Cognitive Behavioral Therapy," *Merriam-Webster's Online Medical Dictionary*, https://www.merriam--webster.com/dictionary/cognitive%20behavioral%20therapy#medicalDictionary. Accessed March 21, 2017.

11. Antonia N. Kaczkurkin and Edna B. Foa, "Cognitive-Behavioral Therapy for Anxiety Disorders: An Update on the Empirical Evidence," *Dialogues in Clinical Neuroscience* 17, no. 3 (September 2015): 337–346, https://www.ncbi.nlm.nih.gov/pmc/articles/PMC4610618/. Accessed March 21, 2017.

Bibliography

"Grit," *Merriam-Webster's Online Dictionary*. Accessed March 21, 2017. https://www.merriam-webster. com/dictionary/grit

"Cognitive Behavioral Therapy," *Merriam-Webster's Online Medical Dictionary*. Accessed March 21, 2017 https://www.merriam-webster.com/dictionary/cognitive%20behavioral%20therapy#medicalDictionary. Accessed March 21, 2017.

Alexander, Ronald. "The Power of Affirmations: How to Make Them Work for You." *Huffington Post*, October 9, 2011. http://www.huffingtonpost.com/ronald-alexander-phd/positive-affirmations_b_921184. html. Accessed March 21, 2017.

Cherry, Kendra. "Psychology—What Are the Id, Ego, and Superego? The Structural Model of Personality." *Very Well*. Last accessed. https://www.verywell.com/the-id-ego-and-superego-2795951. Accessed March 23, 2017.

Ehrlich, Steven D. "Mind-Body Medicine." *University of Maryland Medical Center Medical Reference Guide*. Last accessed. http://umm.edu/health/medical/altmed/treatment/mindbody-medicine. Accessed March 23, 2017.

Gardner, Benjamin. "Making Health Habitual: The Psychology of 'Habit-Formation' and General Practice." *British Journal of General Practice* (December 2012): 664–666. https://www.ncbi.nlm.nih.gov/pmc/articles/PMC3505409/. Accessed March 23, 2017.

Hechtman, Lily, Dusan Kolar, Amanda Keller, Maria Golfinopoulos, Lucy Cumyn, and Cassidy Syer. "Treatment of Adults with Attention-Deficit/Hyperactivity Disorder." *Neuropsychiatry Disease and Treatment* 4, no. 2 (April 2008): 389–403. https://www.ncbi.nlm.nih.gov/pmc/articles/PMC2518387/. Accessed March 23, 2017.

Kaczkurkin, Antonia N. and Edna B. Foa. "Cognitive-Behavioral Therapy for Anxiety Disorders: An Update on the Empirical Evidence." *Dialogues in Clinical Neuroscience* 17, no. 3 (September 2015): 337–346. https://www.ncbi.nlm.nih.gov/pmc/articles/PMC4610618/. Accessed March 23, 2017.

Seidman, Larry J., Joseph Biederman, Lichen Liang, Eve M. Valera, Michael C. Monuteaux, Ariel Brown, Jonathan Kaiser, Thomas Spencer, Stephen V. Faraone, and Nikos Makris. "Gray Matter Alterations in Adults with Attention-Deficit/Hyperactivity Disorder Identified by Voxel-Based Morphometry." *Biological Psychiatry* 69, no. (9)(May 1, 2011): 857–866. https://www.ncbi.nlm. nih.gov/pmc/articles/PMC3940267/. Accessed March 23, 2017.

Steinbach, A.M. "Neurolinguistic Programming: A Systematic Approach to Change." *Canadian Family Physician* 30 (January 1984): 147–150. https://www.ncbi.nlm.nih.gov/ pmc/articles/PMC2153995/?page=1. Accessed March 23, 2017.

Weir, Kirsten. "What You Need to Know about Willpower: The Psychological Science of Self-Control." *APA.org*. Last accessed. http://www.apa.org/helpcenter/will-power.aspx. Accessed March 23, 2017.

About the Author

Darrell Williams is a medical coder for a New York City hospital. Over the past ten years in the medical field, he has acquired advanced knowledge of human anatomy, physiology, clinical disease processes, pharmacology, and medical terminology as he 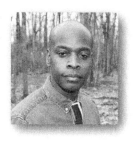 learned about mental health and other diseases together with their clinical application.

In 2016, Darrell was diagnosed with attention-deficit/ hyperactivity disorder (ADHD), which caused him difficulty in performing certain mental tasks. He slowly learned the five secret steps to improving his willpower in order to pursue grit to combat his ADHD. He first practiced these steps in the gym and eventually incorporated them into his everyday life. This is how *In Pursuit of Grit: Five Ways to Transform Your Mind, Develop Your Character and Get the Body You Desire* was created. Darrell's goal is to share these secrets with others so that they can also live up to their fullest potential and not be a casualty of mental disorders, procrastination, laziness, self-doubt, or discouragement.

Made in the USA
Middletown, DE
09 January 2023

21720826R00056